# GENETIC INTERVENTION ON HUMAN SUBJECTS

The Report of a Working Party of
The Catholic Bishops' Joint Committee
on Bioethical Issues

London 1996

Published by
The Catholic Bishops' Joint Committee
on Bioethical Issues

Distributed by
The Linacre Centre
60 Grove End Road
London NW8 9NH

*British Library Cataloguing in Publication Data*

Working Party of the Catholic Bishops'
Joint Committee on Bioethical Issues
  Genetic Intervention on Human Subjects
  1. Title
  174.25

  ISBN 0-9520923-1-X

# Contents

| | |
|---|---|
| Preface | page v |
| Acknowledgements | vii |
| Introduction | 1 |
| Gene therapy: scientific and clinical aspects | 6 |
| Moral considerations: human beings and their fulfilment | 16 |
| The purpose of medicine | 21 |
| Genetic health and genetic responsibility | 24 |
| Genetic interventions: somatic therapy | 28 |
| Genetic interventions: germ-line therapy | 30 |
| Non-therapeutic genetic interventions | 36 |
| Conclusion: permissible forms of genetic intervention | 42 |
| Appendix A: Legal issues (Mr John Duddington) | 45 |
| Appendix B: Extracts from Vatican Documents | 49 |
| Glossary | 56 |
| Bibliography | 62 |
| Notes | 73 |

# Members of the Working Party

| | |
|---|---|
| Dr A.P.Cole KHS FRCP(E) DCH (*Chairman*) | Consultant Paediatrician, Worcester Royal Infirmary |
| Rev John Berry PhD | Associate Research Fellow The Linacre Centre |
| Mr John Duddington LLB | Director of Legal Studies, Worcester College of Technology |
| Dr Ian Jessiman KSG MA MRCP DCH | General Practitioner, London |
| Dr John McLean MD BSc | Manchester Royal Infirmary |
| Mrs Agneta Sutton MPhil | Research Fellow, Centre for Bioethics and Public Policy |
| Dr Helen Watt PhD (*Secretary*) | Research Fellow, The Linacre Centre |

# Preface

Human genetic engineering has been for some time the subject of a lively public debate. For this reason, it was decided by the Catholic Bishops' Joint Committee on Bioethical Issues to bring together a Working Party so that a contribution to this subject could be made from a Catholic perspective. The Report that follows is the product of a four-year process of collaboration by Working Party members.

The Committee is most grateful to the members of the Working Party for the dedication with which they have pursued their task. Particular thanks are owing to Dr Anthony Cole, the Chairman of the Working Party, for enthusiastically undertaking this work alongside so many other commitments, and to Dr Helen Watt who, as Secretary, did so much work on successive drafts of the text. The Committee would also like to thank the Linacre Centre for making available the services of Dr Watt and another Working Party member, the Reverend Dr John Berry. The Centre has provided important services to the Committee over a number of years.

The Report produced by the Working Party gives a clear account both of the scientific aspects of gene therapy, and of some of the moral problems raised by gene therapy and other genetic interventions. Avoiding both the extremes of uncritical acceptance and uncritical rejection of new technology, the Report puts genetic interventions in the context of respect for human persons as bodily beings. While the Report will be of particular interest to Catholics, it will also be of interest to non-Catholic Christians and, indeed, to non-Christian readers. Similarly, the Report should be of interest not only to experts in the fields of clinical genetics and medical ethics, but to those who are new to one or both fields. The Report will be useful both in explaining the forms of intervention which are now or may in the future be available, and in providing a much-needed framework for discussion of the moral questions they raise.

*Thomas J Cardinal Winning*
Archbishop of Glasgow
Chairman of the Catholic Bishops' Joint Committee
on Bioethical Issues

# Acknowledgements

We gratefully acknowledge the help of members of the Catholic Bishops' Joint Committee on Bioethical Issues who made comments on successive drafts of this Report. Thanks are due in particular to Mr Luke Gormally, Rev John Murphy, Bishop Donal Murray, Rev Peter Jeffery CSSp and Professor Peter Millard. We are also grateful for the assistance of Rev Brian Johnstone CSSR of the Lateran University, Rev Anthony Fisher OP of the Australian Catholic University and that of four experts who gave oral evidence to the Working Party: Professor Robert Williamson, formerly of the University of London, and Professor David Morton, Professor Maj Huylten and Dr Heather Draper of the University of Birmingham Departments of Genetics and Biomedical Science and Biomedical Ethics. We also wish to thank Dr Teresa Iglesias of University College, Dublin, Dr John Tolmie, Consultant Clinical Geneticist at the Guthrie Institute, Glasgow, and Dr Tony Tarragona of the Advanced Biotechnology Centre, Charing Cross and Westminster Medical School, London, for their helpful comments on earlier drafts of the Report.

# 1

# Introduction

Clinical genetics is the application of human genetics to the understanding and treatment of genetic disorders. It is an area of rapid expansion; an area in which new information and new skills are constantly accumulating. It is widely hoped that as the nineteenth and twentieth centuries have been successful in combating infectious diseases, subsequent centuries will be successful in combating genetic diseases[1] – the 'last frontier' of medicine.

It must be emphasized that the ability to diagnose genetic disorders at present far exceeds the ability to treat them. In the case of prenatal diagnosis in particular, abortion is by far the most common form of intervention offered if the foetus is found to be affected. However, it is also true that there is, in some cases, the option of using knowledge gained through diagnosis – whether diagnosis of the unborn child or of the older human individual – to make possible earlier and more effective treatment of the condition identified.

The use of gene therapy to correct defects or mitigate their consequences is not, at present, a feasible option in the majority of cases. However, it is widely anticipated that gene therapy will become a more common form of treatment of genetic disorders in the future.

Consider (for example) a couple who discover, when their child is born with **cystic fibrosis**★, that they are carriers of the **gene** which causes this disorder. Cystic fibrosis, the most common genetic disorder among Caucasians, is characterized by abnormal secretions of mucus in the lungs, causing chronic lung infections with eventual destruction of lung tissue. Other manifestations include impaired absorption of nutrients and liver disease; for these, however, there are established treatments. A person born with cystic fibrosis may expect to live for 30–40 years with increasing pulmonary complications.

Cystic fibrosis is an **autosomal recessive** disorder; i.e., it is not sex-linked, and occurs when both parents carry the abnormal gene. In the unlikely event that a child was born to parents both of whom were themselves affected by Cystic fibrosis, or were affected by the gene in other ways[2], that child would also be affected. In contrast, where the parents are merely carriers, on average one in four of their children will be affected in some way.

What should be the response of the parents to the news that they are carriers for cystic fibrosis? The question is important not only for the parents themselves, but for those – such as doctors, counsellors and clergy – to whom the parents may turn for advice. To begin with, what are the options currently available among which the parents must make a morally defensible choice?

The parents may decide not to have another child, and to use sterilization, contraception or natural family planning as a

---

★ Terms explained in the Glossary are printed in bold on their first occurrence in the text.

means of avoiding conception. They may decide to conceive again, but to make use of prenatal diagnosis during any future pregnancy, with a view to aborting the unborn child if he or she has cystic fibrosis. Rarely, they may be offered the new technique of pre-implantation diagnosis after *in vitro* fertilisation, so that affected embryos may be rejected for the purpose of implantation. There are, however, serious moral questions, of varying degrees of importance, raised by almost all these options. In particular, the last two options, which allow for the intentional destruction of the affected unborn child, are in this way radically destructive of the parent-child relationship, in making parental acceptance conditional on the child's state of health.

What are the other options available to parents confronting – perhaps with considerable sorrow and anxiety – the fact that they are carriers? The parents may decide to accept the risk of having another child with cystic fibrosis, taking into account the value inherent in the life of the child they now have, and the life of the child they may have in the future. In making this decision, they may also take into consideration new possibilities of treatment which may in the future be available.

Such possibilities include a form of treatment which is now under trial: **somatic** gene therapy, by which the correct gene is introduced into the affected part of the patient – in this case, the respiratory tract. Somatic therapy affects only the individual on whom it is carried out, and not that individual's descendants. There is, however, a remote possibility that at some time in the future **germ-line** gene therapy on **gametes** or on embryos might ensure that descendants of the individual treated would be born without the defective gene. While it is likely that germ-line gene therapy would be carried out in the context of *in vitro* fertilization, germ-line therapy can also be envisaged in the context of natural procreation.

Gene therapy is usually thought of in connection with *inherited* diseases. However, the main applications of gene therapy will probably lie in improving the treatment of *acquired* diseases, such as AIDS and cancer. In the case of cancer, somatic gene therapy could be used to elicit immune responses to cancer cells, or to modify tumour tissue in order to enhance the effectiveness of chemotherapy. It should be added that increasing knowledge of the genetic factors involved in disease is likely to make possible a more effective use of conventional medicine without recourse to gene therapy.

## *Outline of this Report*

In this Report, we examine some of the moral, legal, scientific and clinical issues raised by gene therapy and other genetic interventions. The Report is addressed not only to those readers who have an academic interest in these issues but to those who find themselves (or may in the future find themselves) confronted with these issues in the course of their work in areas such as science, law, medicine and pastoral care. It is also addressed to those readers who have a more personal interest in these issues, because they are themselves affected by genetic disorders and/or because they have or might have children who are affected by genetic disorders. In view of the fact that gene therapy is still under trial, and is not available for the great majority of patients, we have sought to place gene therapy very much within the context of clinical genetics as it is currently practised.

The Report begins with a brief scientific account of gene therapy, and of the disorders for which it has been tried or is being considered. There follows an attempt to provide a philosophical and theological background to the moral evaluation of gene therapy and other genetic interventions. After looking in turn at somatic and germ-line therapy, we devote some attention to the morality of non-therapeutic genetic interventions. The conclusion summarizes the findings of the Working Party with regard to somatic and germ-line therapy and other interventions which are or could be made on the basis of genetic information.

# 2

# Gene therapy: scientific and clinical aspects[3]

Gene therapy is the intentional alteration of genes in cells or tissues in such a way as to treat or prevent an inherited disorder, or to make another pathological condition more amenable to treatment.

Such intervention is termed *somatic* gene therapy if the alteration affects only the individual on whom it is carried out. If the intervention takes place on the germ-line cells – that is, sperm, ova or their precursors – it is termed *germ-line* gene therapy, and will affect not only a particular individual but also his or her descendants.

The consensus among scientists is that germ-line therapy is unethical, at least in our current state of knowledge. This chapter will deal not with germ-line, but with somatic gene therapy, which has already been carried out on patients in a range of clinical trials.

## Background Genetics

### Chromosomes

Each human cell, except the mature red blood cell, has a nucleus which contains the **chromosomes**. The units of genetic information, the genes, are arranged in a linear fashion along the chromosomes in the form of the chemical **DNA** (deoxyribonucleic acid). The human species has a characteristic **karyotype**, or number and type of chromosomes, and each gene (except for 'jumping genes') has a precise position or **locus** on a particular chromosome.

Genes which have their loci on the same chromosome are described as linked or syntenic. The alternative forms of a gene which may occupy the same locus are called **alleles**. Although each chromosome bears only a single allele at a given locus, there may be multiple alleles for that locus in the general population. The **genotype** is the individual's genetic constitution – usually described with reference to the specific allele at one particular locus – while the **phenotype** is the **expression** of that genotype in the structure or physiology of the individual.

Human cells are divided into two types: somatic or body cells and germ-line cells which are set aside in the embryonic sex organs to provide ova or sperm. Normal somatic cells contain 46 chromosomes: 23 matched, or homologous pairs. One chromosome of each pair is inherited from the father, the other from the mother, and one of each pair will be transmitted to the children of the person whose chromosomes they are.

The chromosomes in each pair have the same gene loci in the same sequence, and at any one locus they may have either the same or different alleles. 22 of the chromosome pairs are termed autosomes and are identified individually by number (1,2,3...22). The remaining pair are the sex chromosomes and are designated XX in the female and XY in the male. The normal female karyotype is 46XX and that of the male is 46XY. The karyotype of a female child with **Down's**

**Syndrome** will be expressed 47XX + 21, indicating that there is an additional chromosome 21 present.

*Cell division*

There are two types of cell division: **mitosis** and **meiosis**. Mitotic division generates two cells which are genetically identical to the single cell from which they originated, and hence each daughter cell possesses the full complement of 46 chromosomes. This process of mitosis is the means by which the single cell embryo generates an estimated $10^{14}$ cells all of which are genetically identical in the mature human being.

Meiosis is a division which occurs only in the ovaries and testes and results in the production of germ-line cells each of which possesses only 23 chromosomes. Thus when an ovum is fertilised by a sperm the resulting single cell embryo has 46 chromosomes – 23 inherited from the father and 23 from the mother.

*DNA*

Each of the 46 chromosomes is made up of DNA which takes the form of a double stranded helix. Attached to each strand of the helix is a series of alternating nucleotides, often known as **bases**. The four bases are adenine (A), guanine (G), cytosine (C) and thymine (T). The strands of the helix are held together, like the strands of a rope-ladder, by the chemical bonds which form between the bases. A bonds only with T and G only with C, so that if a sequence of bases on one strand is ATGCCAG the sequence on the other strand will be its mirror image: TACGGTC. It is this sequence of bases on either strand which constitutes a gene, providing information which will eventually be used for the manufacture of proteins in the cell.

When chromosomes **replicate** during cell division (mitosis) the two strands of DNA separate along their length and each strand acts as a template for the synthesis of a new strand. Each new double helix contains one of the original strands, together with a new strand which has been constructed on the basis of the information found on the original strand.

*Transcription and translation*

The cell contains another nucleic acid which is present both in the nucleus and outside it in the cytoplasm. This is ribonucleic acid or **RNA**, which unlike DNA is single stranded, and has the base uracil (U) in place of thymine (T).

RNA has several functions within the cell, one of its most important being as messenger RNA or mRNA. The role of mRNA is to transfer genetic information contained as DNA within the nucleus into the cytoplasm of the cell. There it will be used to direct the production of proteins which determine the function of that cell or tissue.

The conversion of DNA into RNA is a process called **transcription**. This process involves a specific sequence of bases in the DNA of a chromosome – the sequence containing the gene to be transcribed. Over that sequence, the strands of DNA separate, and a strand of RNA is synthesized using one of the strands as a template. When the strands of DNA come back together, the RNA is released from the chromosome. Thereafter it undergoes a 'splicing' procedure which removes non-informative sequences of bases and splices together informative sequences to form mature mRNA. When splicing is complete, the mRNA leaves the nucleus to enter the surrounding space in the cell, in order to direct the production of proteins by the process of **translation**.

The gene remains in the nucleus, sending messages outside the nucleus whenever more protein is needed by the cell. Some genes will be activated and other genes silenced, depending on what is needed by the part of the body which will be affected.

*Mutations*

For genetic information to be reliably present in the cells, there needs to be an extremely accurate mechanism for DNA replication before cell division, and a mechanism for repairing the many accidental changes that occur in DNA. Should this repair process fail, a permanent change or mutation is introduced into the DNA. The phenotypic effect of a mutation on the individual human being depends on the site of the mutation, and the alteration it induces in any gene product. A faulty gene containing the wrong sequence of bases may result in a missing or faulty protein and in a serious genetic disorder.

*Recombinant DNA Technology*

With the recognition that both DNA replication and the genetic code were founded on sequences of bases, research activity was focussed on sequencing the bases in DNA. The co-operative work of scientists throughout the world on the location of genes on chromosomes and the definition of their chemical structures is known as the **Human Genome Project**.

Genes can be spliced into (for example) a bacterial chromosome; the bacteria then multiply and produce vast numbers of copies of the gene, which can be studied by scientists. The isolated gene can be inserted into living cells cultivated in the laboratory, which then produce the protein for which the inserted gene carries the code. Proteins can be produced in this way and made available for therapeutic use; for example, insulin for the treatment of diabetes.

## *Medical applications of the new technology*

The new technology has provided more specific tests for many diseases. It has also been used in the production of effective vaccines against infectious diseases, such as Hepatitis B. Its use to produce proteins absent in certain genetic diseases has also been valuable. However, a more appropriate solution to genetic diseases would be to insert a copy of the gene for the absent protein into those cells which would normally express that gene as the protein product. Ideally, the defective gene would be replaced by the normal copy at the same site on the genome; however, this would be more difficult than the random insertion of the normal gene.

A number of different gene delivery systems are being developed, and clinical trials of their efficacy in the treatment of several disorders have begun. Such an approach has much to offer, not only in the treatment of genetic diseases but also as a means of introducing into cancer cells genes for specific target **antigens** which will halt the growth of tumours.

The situation with regard to genetic disease, however, is even more complex than it might seem. A mutation in a structural gene, i.e. one that codes for a protein, will affect the expression of that protein. However, failure of expression may occur in the presence of a normal structural gene because of a mutation in one of the control genes which regulate which genes will be 'switched on' and which will be 'switched off'. There is much that remains to be discovered as to how these control genes work. Similarly, it is difficult to understand why, in an autosomal **dominant** condition such as **Huntington's Chorea**, the presence of a defective gene prevents the function of the intact allele on the other chromosome.

## Gene therapy: delivery systems

Effective gene therapy requires the recognition and isolation of the appropriate gene, together with an efficient delivery system or **vector**. Vectors must be non-toxic and able to target the appropriate cell population. The DNA they introduce must be transcriptionally active, non-disruptive and able to express the gene product at adequate levels for long enough to correct the disease.

### Vectors

Genes can be inserted into cells directly by physical techniques or by using a biological vector for delivery. Viruses can be used as vectors, in view of their natural tendency to enter cells and insert their genome into the genome of the cell. The healthy human gene is inserted into the virus genome, with the hope that it will then be delivered by the virus into the human genome.

One illness for which virus vectors have been used is cystic fibrosis. The adenovirus which naturally targets human lungs has been used to carry the gene for the protein whose absence causes chest infections and eventual lung damage in children with cystic fibrosis. However, there is some concern as to the possible dangers of using adenovirus vectors when repeated exposure is required to maintain a therapeutic effect. Until this anxiety is resolved, such vectors appear to be more suited to short-term therapy.

*Other methods of delivery*

There are other, non-biological methods by which genes can be delivered to cells. DNA can be placed in artificial **lipid vesicles**, or fatty bubbles, which fuse with the membranes of human cells so that the DNA can enter those cells. Direct injection of naked DNA into tumours has also been shown to result in gene transfer and expression, often with an efficiency which may be of therapeutic benefit.

The main advantage of these methods is that they impose few constraints on the size or sequence length of the gene inserted. In addition they avoid the incorporation of viral sequences which may be hazardous to the patient. In the case of lipid vesicles it would, however, be desirable to develop techniques for more precise targeting by attaching to the vesicles an antibody which would recognize the target cells.

## *Gene therapy: clinical trials and possibilities*

An expanding number of conditions are now being treated by somatic gene therapy. However, there is some dispute as to whether trials to date have shown a beneficial clinical effect. While it does not seem as if there have been serious *negative* effects from trials of somatic gene therapy, the benefits of such trials have been contested, and there is, in any case, a lack of published results in this area.[4]

The first inherited disease to be treated by gene therapy was **adenosine deaminase (ADA) deficiency**.[5] This disease involves a congenital immune abnormality of certain bone marrow cells, which can lead to recurrent infections. Although gene therapy appeared to show a beneficial result, it is difficult to tell to what extent this was due to the conventional treatment which the subjects of the trial were also receiving.[6]

In the case of cystic fibrosis, mice have been genetically altered so that they manifest this disease hitherto only known in man. They have been used as experimental models, and clinical trials with genetically altered adenoviruses to reverse the cystic fibrosis gene abnormality have taken place in Britain and the U.S.[7]

Other diseases caused by single gene defects may also become susceptible to treatment in time. These include **muscular dystrophy**, **haemophilia** and **chronic granulomatous disease**. It is not yet apparent how DNA can be inserted into the tissues affected by these diseases in a way that would permit it consistently to express its corrective effect.

The first application of somatic gene therapy in non inherited diseases will be in the treatment of a number of cancers.[8] Cells are removed from tumours and by genetic modification their immunosensitivity is altered. By returning these cells to the body a strong antibody reaction takes place destroying these and the other comparable cancer cells. Some of the first cancers so treated include the previously incurable hepatocellular carcinomas.[9]

The Human Immunodeficiency Virus (HIV) which causes AIDS may be genetically influenced and rendered more liable to the action of such therapeutic agents as Interferon. The HIV infected **lymphocytes** are altered to render them susceptible to this substance.[10]

Even a metabolic disease such as insulin dependent diabetes may be treatable by somatic gene therapy. The insulin **receptors** may be altered by the transfer of genetically altered **lipoproteins**. There has already been some *in vitro* alteration of cells both in animals and in man.[11]

Genes express themselves via a number of intermediary stages until they produce their final outcome, a single protein.

Identification of the gene and an understanding of how it will express itself opens up possibilities of blocking expression at various points with new therapeutic interventions. The pharmaceutical industry is actively engaged in fundamental research in this area.

# 3

# Moral Considerations: Human beings and their fulfilment

We have looked at some of the scientific aspects of somatic gene therapy. What are the moral implications of gene therapy and other genetic interventions? Before attempting to answer this question, we need to ask more fundamental questions concerning the nature of human beings and the ways in which we are fulfilled. We need to ask, more specifically, what is the role of medicine in promoting our fulfilment, and what are our general responsibilities with regard to the genetic health of ourselves and our children.

A human being is not a purely spiritual entity, but a being at once spiritual and physical – *corpore et anima unus*. I am not a mere soul, even if my soul survives death. Rather, I am a biological being – an animal – sharing biological characteristics with non-human animals, but in a way that is fully human. My biological nature is not 'subpersonal', not something separate than what I am myself; rather, it has the moral importance of the nature of a human person.

The unity of the human person can be explained by reference to the role of the soul as the body's 'life-principle': that by which the body is made alive.[12] On this understanding, a living human body cannot exist without a human soul. The question of when a human person, with a human soul, comes into existence can thus be equated with the question of when the living human organism – the living human 'whole' – comes into being. On current evidence, the human 'whole' appears to originate at fertilization in the majority of cases, although in the case of identical twinning he or she may originate by later asexual reproduction.

The fulfilment or flourishing of the human being as the kind of being he or she is has been the subject of renewed interest among a number of contemporary philosophers. A particular approach we have found helpful[13] refers to *basic human goods*, in respect of which human beings are said to flourish as the personal beings they are. Among such goods is the good of life, in its transmission, health and safety. Knowledge and some degree of excellence in work and play constitute other basic goods. In addition, harmony with others, and with God, the ultimate source of our being, are included in this account of human goods.

### The good of life and health

To be fulfilled in our existence as human beings requires some degree of bodily well-being. Health is a good which is a dimension of the basic good of life. It should be understood as some measure of ability to function well both physically and mentally, beyond the basic functional ability required for life itself. The good of health is both a *basic* human good – a good in itself – and an *instrumental* good which makes it possible to participate in goods such as knowledge and friendship.

### Respect for human goods: positive and negative requirements

Moral principles are concerned with human fulfilment – with the enjoyment of human goods. At any time they exist, human beings or 'persons'[14] have morally significant interests in all the human goods in which they may eventually participate. Thus not only the infant, but the foetus and the embryo have morally significant interests in knowledge and friendship, as well as in the good of life and health. There are, however, moral constraints – for example, those concerning the interests of others – on the ways in which the interests of human beings may be promoted. The life and health of some may not be promoted by means of an attack on innocent others; for example, by means of destructive experimentation on human subjects. More generally, it is not morally required – nor even possible, in view of limited resources – to go to all conceivable lengths to promote the life of every human being. The duty to *promote* life, unlike the duty *not to attack* the lives of innocent human beings, does not apply in every situation.

### *Respect for life: the Christian tradition*

From a Christian perspective, life can be seen not simply as a basic human good, but as a gift from God. All human beings share the same origin and are called to the same destiny: to find happiness with God for all eternity. Unlike other creatures, human beings have the radical capacity[15] for rational behaviour whose ultimate realization is friendship with God. The right of all human beings to be respected is founded on this radical capacity.

Respect for human beings requires respect for their interests in the basic human goods, including the good of life, or human bodily existence. As a gift from God, life is to be valued and (in many situations) promoted, and is never – at least in the case of *innocent* life – to be deliberately attacked.

Life must not only be respected where it is already present; it must be respected in its transmission. The procreation of human life is a mission or vocation which, on the Christian understanding, belongs to married couples, who are called to a love which is naturally ordered to the gift of new life. By means of an act expressive of marital union, the couple are given the power to initiate a process which may be completed by the action of God in creating a new human person.

The Catholic Church in particular teaches that the couple should be willing to receive and welcome, as a gift from God, any child who may result from their freely chosen intercourse. The couple may choose, for good reasons, not to have intercourse at times they know they will be fertile, but should make no attempt to make otherwise fertile intercourse infertile.[16] Similarly, the couple should only attempt to have children by means of normal marital intercourse.[17] While a doctor may *assist* the process begun by marital intercourse to end in conception, it is not permissible to *replace* marital intercourse by an act of production, or control over materials, as in (for example) *in vitro* fertilization.[18] Husband and wife are non-substitutable in what belongs to their marriage: sexual union leading to the procreation, with God, of new human life.

Children conceived as the result of an act with this kind of dignity are more likely to be accepted unconditionally after their conception than children who have come into being as 'products of a making' – by means of technical control over biological materials.[19] Thus *in vitro* fertilization will normally involve the production of a number of embryos, after which 'spare' or 'defective' embryos will be frozen, discarded or used in destructive experimentation. IVF couples and donors will normally have consented to this kind of 'quality control' and 'use' of their embryos. Their attitude of *domination* over what are – whether or not they know this – their children is incompatible with responsible parenthood, and with respect for young human beings.

However, even in a case in which an IVF child was respected unconditionally after his or her conception, the way in which conception was brought about *in vitro* would not be appropriate to a human person. The child conceived through a production process geared to meeting the wishes of the parents comes into being as a product – and thus in a symbolically subordinate relation to the parents – even if the parents accept that the child is a person equal in dignity to themselves. In contrast, where the child is *received* by the parents as an outcome of marital self-giving, he or she embodies an *interpersonal act of love*, not a wish to produce what the parents want. Such a child is not a manifestation of an act of domination over persons or materials to produce some desired effect, but is rather a manifestation of the parents' unconditional acceptance both of each other and of the child they do, in fact, conceive.

# 4

# The purpose of medicine

How should we understand the purpose of medicine, in the light of the principles outlined in the previous chapter? Medicine is a form of activity concerned with the promotion of the basic good of health. The patient, who is unable to promote his or her health unaided, entrusts him or herself to the doctor in the hope of achieving what cannot otherwise be achieved. Medicine is concerned with the management of the patient for the purpose of combating some functional disorder and the effects of this disorder, either through prevention, through cure, or (in the case of palliative treatment) through the relief of pain and distress. Medicine is concerned with involuntary shortcomings in the functional contribution made by the parts of the human being to the good of the whole.

Medicine exists to serve *health* — that is, the complex of *functional, goal-directed psychophysical systems* (hereafter, **teleologies**), all of which are valuable in the contribution they make to the good of the whole. For example, the capacity to take food manually, swallow and digest it is a normal human capacity; it would be wrong for a doctor to deprive a healthy person of this capacity, even if the person could then be fed in some alternative way. Medicine does not replace or supplement human teleologies on an arbitrary basis, but rather attempts to restore them, or (in conjunction with nursing) to make up for their absence or failure. As far as possible, medicine works *with* human teleologies; for example, with the natural ability of the human body to heal itself and fight infection. However, medical interventions are an attempt to make up for the absence of healthy teleologies – and thus are frequently, to some extent, 'imposed' on the patient who passively accepts them.

If there is a value both to the *presence* and to the *use* of human functions in promoting human well-being, then externally imposed interventions, while they may be necessary and good, are to some degree lacking in this value. In general, human fulfilment is best promoted through the normal channels of human *activity*, whether conscious or non-conscious. However, externally imposed interventions can sometimes be justified on the grounds that the usual means to self-fulfilment, on the basis of healthy human functions, are for some reason unavailable, or unsatisfactory. *Medical*, as opposed to (for example) *cosmetic* interventions are justified in terms of a need to respond to some *involuntary*[20] *functional defect* of the human being. It is the need to respond to such a defect which marks off medicine from other attempts to benefit human beings.

It is therefore the purpose of medicine to meet a need created by some functional defect, or by the possibility of some functional defect, either by curative or preventative treatment, or by the palliation of symptoms. Medicine is concerned with 'health' not in the broad sense, which refers to a very high level of psychophysical capacity[21], but in a more precise sense, which refers to a more modest level of such capacity. Thus a certain level of health can be achieved by (for example) a person in chronic pain, who may be able to participate in various human goods despite being far removed from a position of general psychophysical well-being.

It should go without saying that it is no part of the purpose of medicine to *harm* a human being, by such means as destructive experimentation. Nor is it part of the purpose of medicine to expose a human being to excessive *risks* of harm. In the words of the Declaration of Helsinki, 'Concern for the interests of the subject must always prevail over the interest of science and society'.[22]

# 5

# Genetic health and genetic responsibility

Health is not simply the concern of the doctor, but the concern of the competent patient, who is responsible for taking care of his or her mental and physical well-being. Health is the result of an interaction between an individual's structure – both genetic and non-genetic – and his or her environment, including other human beings. This interaction will often be influenced by the individual's choices, and those of other people. It is unreasonable to focus solely on the influence on health of structural features such as genes, without taking into account the many environmental and social factors which influence health, and for which human beings may be responsible.

The responsibility of the competent person for his or her health includes a responsibility for his or her *genetic* health – both in so far as it affects the individual and in so far as it affects his or her descendants.[23] Part of what is involved in responsible parenthood is the taking of reasonable steps to prevent genetic damage to one's children – for example, by avoiding excessive exposure to radiation. In view of the fact that damage to gametes may have an impact beyond the next generation to all subsequent generations, potential parents must be thought of as having some kind of responsibility with regard to the health of even their remote descendants.

On the question of responsibility for the health of one's children and more remote descendants, it should be noted that there is no 'blanket right' to have a child – or even to try to have a child by means of normal marital intercourse. The right of married couples to try to have children will depend on the situation in which they find themselves placed. For example, a man affected by radiation may have a duty to wait until the risks of genetic damage are lowered before he tries to have a child. A couple who find that they are carriers for some serious genetic disorder may sometimes have a duty to take morally acceptable steps to avoid conception altogether. They may have this duty, for example, if they are not in a position to meet the needs of a child with that disorder themselves, with the reasonable assistance of society.[24]

However, the decision to conceive or not to conceive a child who will or may have some genetic disorder is one which must be made by the couple themselves, without undue influence, on the basis of morally relevant information. Moreover, it should be noted that if a couple are entitled – in some cases even obliged – to seek to avoid conception, whether on genetic grounds or on such grounds as family poverty, this is quite compatible with their recognition of the intrinsic, 'core' value of the life of the child they might otherwise conceive. The couple are, or should be, seeking to avoid certain disvalues, such as the unmet needs of the child, rather than judging that the child, if conceived, would not be a human being whose life had the fundamental value of any human life.

Part of what is meant by the 'equality' of human beings – that is, their 'equality in dignity' – is the fundamental, intrinsic value of every human life. Whatever *subjective* value a life may have to an individual and to his or her family, the individual's life has *objective* value as the life of a human being. To say that human beings are equal in their basic human dignity is to say, first, that the bodily existence of all human beings is objectively good, and secondly, that all human beings have morally significant interests – which may be fulfilled to a greater or lesser extent – in health and in other human goods. To whatever extent an individual can participate in health and other human goods, the good of his or her life precludes an attempt on this life on the grounds that it is worthless.[25]

With regard to the suffering – of the child and of the parents – which may accompany the birth of a disabled child, it must be acknowledged that suffering is in itself an evil, and therefore something human beings are often justified in seeking to prevent. However, it is a common human experience that suffering – which is, in some degree, widespread in the lives of human beings – can provide an occasion for what is genuinely good. Certainly, it is the experience of many parents of disabled children that whatever suffering may accompany the lives of these children, their lives are of value both in themselves and in the impact they have on the rest of the family. The most severely disabled can draw attention, by their sheer presence, to the value of humanity itself: to the radical equality in dignity of all members of the human family.

It is worth remembering that human beings are all imperfect in a variety of ways, and that genetic disease in particular will never be eliminated, as new mutations are occurring all the time. It is also worth remembering that the attitudes of others are influential in making a disability – a functional disorder – a major handicap in the society in which the disabled person lives. The appropriate response to the possibility or presence of some genetic disorder will often be to alter the environment of the individual who will or may be affected. In particular, the appropriate response to the burdens disability can place on the disabled person's family will often be to assist the family with that person's care.

Of course, the provision of care for the disabled can involve the State in considerable financial costs. However, a certain level of such care, in an affluent society such as Britain, is morally required. Certainly, the signs which are visible from time to time of a financial interest on the part of the State in promoting prenatal screening give cause for serious concern.[26]

In view of the variety of uses, both good and bad, to which genetic information can be put, it is vital that such information be conveyed to those seeking it, including parents and potential parents, within a sound ethical framework. If possible, parents and potential parents should be given the opportunity to meet a child with the relevant disorder; at any rate, the counsellor should guard against presenting an unduly negative picture of life with that disorder.

In view of the fact that the rights of disabled children are often threatened in connection with prenatal diagnosis in particular,[27] genetic counsellors should be given some form of training in advocacy on behalf of the disabled. Indeed, it can be argued that genetic counsellors should not merely be *encouraged*, but *required* to have some experience outside a clinical context of working with the disabled and their families.

# 6

# Genetic interventions: somatic therapy

Assuming an attitude of respect towards those affected by genetic disorders, what should be said about somatic gene therapy? As a response to the medical needs of the patient, we do not believe that somatic therapy is different in principle from other forms of medical treatment. Somatic therapy involves invasive measures targeting organs and tissues of individual patients. It affects the individual alone (or at least, it is not *aimed* at affecting anyone else[28]). The moral questions raised by somatic therapy are therefore similar to those raised by other forms of therapy, and concern the potential benefits to the patient, the risks to the patient and to others[29], and the cost and other burdens of the treatment.

As with any other experimental form of treatment, there is a case for saying that somatic gene therapy should be used, at least at first, to treat cases of serious disease where there is no satisfactory alternative treatment.[30] More generally, somatic therapy should meet the standard moral requirements for experimental therapy. Research should be competently performed and the results audited and assessed by independent bodies; there should be informed consent on the part of the subject, or the parent or guardian in the case of those not able to give consent; there should be proportionality between the risks and burdens of the treatment and the degree and likelihood of benefit.

## Legal restrictions on genetic interventions

There are legal, as well as moral, restrictions on the activities of those who carry out somatic therapy and other genetic interventions. In the case of professional incompetence, the doctor could be sued for damages by the subject. The doctor could also face civil or criminal charges if the appropriate consent on the part of the subject or his or her parent or guardian had not been obtained before the intervention was carried out. For a more detailed discussion of the legal questions raised by genetic interventions, see Appendix A to this Report.

# 7

# Genetic interventions: germ-line therapy

The case of germ-line therapy is very much more complex than that of somatic therapy, partly – but not exclusively – due to the fact that germ-line therapy aims at affecting an indefinite number of people. It is difficult to be clear about just what may be a realistic possibility in this area: the information available seems contradictory and far from certain. However, what is clear is the greater technical difficulty of germ-line therapy, and the increased number of moral questions raised by such therapy.

The practical difficulties of germ-line therapy are widely agreed to be formidable. Indeed, it is often observed that germ-line therapy would be superfluous, as well as very difficult, wherever there was the possibility of transferring only normal embryos to the uterus after *in vitro* fertilization. In a society in which it is seen as appropriate to eliminate disease by eliminating affected individuals, *selection* of embryos is more likely to become common practice – because simpler and cheaper – than therapy on embryos, or on gametes.

Even if germ-line therapy were thought worth pursuing, in practice both therapy on embryos and therapy on gametes would be very likely to be associated with *in vitro* fertilization or similar techniques, with all the disrespect for human procreation, and for actual human lives, which these techniques involve.[31]

The objections to IVF and similar techniques of non-sexual reproduction would not, of course, apply to the screening of unfertilized ova, so that the couple could seek to conceive by marital intercourse following the replacement of normal ova. Similarly, these objections would not apply to germ-line therapy on ova or **spermatagonia**[32], if this could be followed by normal marital intercourse. It is more difficult to imagine a situation in which germ-line therapy could be carried out on an embryo who had been naturally conceived. Perhaps such therapy could be carried out *in situ* on the post-implantation embryo, or the pre-implantation embryo could be treated *in situ*, or else retrieved from the fallopian tube, treated, and then implanted. In any case, this kind of therapy, like the therapy on gametes and their precursors mentioned earlier, would escape the specific moral objections to non-sexual reproduction.

### *Objections to germ-line therapy: the 'right to an unchanged genetic inheritance'*

What other objections might be raised to germ-line therapy, if it did not involve non-sexual reproduction? It is sometimes argued that human beings have the right to inherit a genome which has not been artificially changed. The human genome is felt by many people to be in some way special: what, in some radical and irreplaceable way we owe to the past and contribute to the future. What we receive genetically is part of what we are as unique individuals who originate from the interaction and bodily union of two other unique individuals. Indeed, it is sometimes suggested that the genome constitutes the individual in some very strong sense, such that he or she would *literally* not be the same individual after a change to his or her genome.

With regard to this last suggestion, while we recognize the importance of the genome in constituting the individual human being, we would not wish to argue that changes to an individual's genome – any more than to some other part of the body – would result in that individual's substitution by what is *literally* someone else. Both genetic damage (such as through radiation) and genetic therapy (such as germ-line therapy) would appear to be changes *to one and the same individual* – always assuming there is a living human being at the end of the process. The uniqueness of an individual is not tied to the retention of a particular genome. And in fact, a particular genome (if not a particular instance of that genome) can be shared by two individuals, in the case of identical twins.

Assuming that the genome is not essential, in every part, to the survival of the human individual, is the genome nonetheless morally 'untouchable' by virtue of its special role in human development? We would argue not, in view of the fact that the genome is simply one highly influential part of our bodies: the part which directs the formation of other parts, both in ourselves and in our offspring. We believe that, like other parts of the body, the genome may *in principle* be altered, to cure some defect of the body. If a person's reproductive potential is in some way faulty, to amend that potential is, in principle, an acceptable means of promoting the health of that person, and of his or her descendants. We can imagine situations in which to choose this kind of treatment would be, not simply a *right* of the person choosing it, but morally required. Granted that people should not be deprived *without good reason* of the genes they would otherwise have inherited from their parents and passed on to their children, the real possibility of eliminating from a family some serious disease – for example, Huntington's Chorea – would appear to be good enough reason to improve on a person's genetic makeup and reproductive potential.

## *Objections to germ-line therapy: consent, risks, costs*

There are, however, other moral questions which arise concerning risks of, costs of, and consent to, germ-line therapy. On the question of consent, while it is permissible sometimes to carry out medical interventions without the permission either of the patient (if he or she is a minor) or of the parent or guardian (if permission is not available) it is certainly preferable to seek permission, other things being equal, if permission is or will be available. However, lack of consent, if it can be overlooked in other areas, could presumably be overlooked in the area of germ-line therapy, in case of similar need on the part of those who would otherwise have been affected by a serious genetic disease.

Where we find the major problem in accepting germ-line therapy is in the risks such therapy would, in practice, pose to those involved. Quite apart from the risks to the woman which would accompany IVF and/or therapy on ova, the risks to the embryo of germ-line therapy would be considerable, at least at the present stage of technology. Animal experiments have shown a high level of mortality and morbidity in embryos subjected to germ-line interventions. While a relatively high risk for the subject of medical intervention can sometimes be justified in the case of a particularly serious disease, the current risks to the embryo of germ-line interventions – whether on the embryo or on the gametes which form it – go beyond what is reasonable.

In addition to these substantial short-term risks, there is the risk of adversely affecting the germ-line, causing undesired hereditary side-effects, which might be difficult to undo. In order for germ-line therapy to work, the genes would have to be expressed in the right way, in the right tissues of the body; unsuccessful germ-line therapy could cause lasting damage in disrupting the operation of normal genes.[33] There is widespread agreement among scientists that germ-line therapy is, at least at present, too dangerous to contemplate; hence the international moratorium on this kind of intervention.

Whether or not germ-line therapy will *ever* be sufficently safe to consider is, of course, a different question. If experimentation on animals[34] – perhaps in conjunction with computer modelling – could yield sufficient information to make possible experimental *therapy* on humans, we can imagine a situation in which the risks of such therapy would be justified, at least in the case of an otherwise fatal disease. However, it must be remembered that those at risk from such therapy would include those family members who would have been unaffected by the disease in question – assuming they would have existed at all. Moreover, there is a very real question whether the costs of developing and carrying out such therapy could be justified, given the other claims on medical resources. In most cases, germ-line therapy would not be a means of treating those who would have existed whether or not this treatment was available; rather, it would be a means of treating those who were only conceived *because* this treatment was available. It would be harder to justify either the costs or the risks of germ-line therapy where it was not a case of treating an individual, and his or her descendants, who would have existed whether or not germ-line therapy had been offered to that individual's parents.

Moreover, it is likely that even if germ-line therapy *did* become sufficiently safe and affordable at some time in the future, this would be not (or not only) due to animal experimentation, but to experimentation on human embryos. Even after germ-line therapy had been developed, it is likely that, in most cases, the embryo and foetus who had been subjected to such therapy without success would be discarded or aborted. To choose to undergo a therapy which had been developed, and was still performed, in the case of other patients, at such a cost in human life would be to risk the appearance of condoning such treatment of young human beings. This is not to say that to accept such therapy, especially where it was already standard medical treatment, would necessarily be immoral. The parents could, after all, make it clear that they would only consent to germ-line therapy on the understanding that no embryo was harmed, whether or not the treatment was successful. However, the risk of seeming to condone the means by which the therapy was developed, together with the potential witness to the sanctity of life[35] in refusing to accept such a therapy, would be among the factors to be taken into consideration in deciding whether or not to accept it.

# 8

# Non-therapeutic genetic interventions

It may be asked, finally, whether *non-therapeutic* genetic changes, either somatic or germ-line, could ever be justified, if they were sufficiently safe. It must be said at the outset that it is doubtful that non-therapeutic genetic interventions will ever be sufficiently safe to consider. Certainly, this must be said of germ-line interventions, which are currently far too hazardous even for *therapeutic* purposes.

Many features which people might desire for themselves or their children – for example, increased intelligence – involve a number of genes as well as environmental factors, such that there would be enormous problems in attempting to confer these features by genetic means. Most non-therapeutic genetic interventions belong, for the forseeable future, to the realm of science fiction. There is, however, something to be gained by asking what kind of non-therapeutic genetic interventions might *in principle* be justified, as the discussion of this brings up more general questions concerning structural interventions on human beings.

### *Attempts to produce a change which is not objectively beneficial.*

Non-therapeutic interventions which are not 'perfective', but merely cause permanent disruption to normal human functioning, are morally unacceptable.[36] It is actively harmful to deprive a person of some existing function, or to provide a function not possessed by normal human beings, except in so far as this will promote that person's interests – for example, protect him or her against disease.[37] As a *minimum*, those who perform an intervention which disrupts an individual's normal functioning must want to confer what is objectively a benefit – for example, by reinforcing that or another function.

What is at stake is not simply consent on the part of the subject of intervention. For even if the subject *does* consent to some non-therapeutic, non-perfective intervention, this fact alone does not justify this kind of intervention. Neither medicine nor any other area of worthwhile human activity is simply about giving people what they want, whether for others or themselves. Rather, medicine, and other worthwhile activities, are concerned with the promotion of human well-being.

### *Attempts to produce a change which is objectively beneficial*

What should we say about attempts to produce 'perfective'[38] changes in the individual, or in the germ-line: changes which are objectively beneficial? One might think of those changes, such as increased intelligence, which many parents, in particular, believe they are justified in promoting by non-genetic means such as mental stimulation in early childhood.

We have argued in a previous chapter that human teleological systems, of the kind required for early learning, are in themselves valuable. It is the existence of such functional systems which constitutes the basic good of health. Not only is human teleology in itself valuable, but there is, we believe, a *prima facie* case for *making use* exclusively of human teleology in promoting human well-being. People should not, for example, be tube-fed as a 'healthy alternative' to taking food normally. It is better that people use their capacities more fully by feeding themselves in the normal way.

In other words, we need to have sufficient reason to supplement or bypass the normal means to human fulfilment through our human teleology. Such a reason exists, for example, in the case of *medical need* for such a supplement or bypass: a need created by some pathological defect, such that the normal teleological means to self-fulfilment are not now appropriate.

This is not to say that there are no justified *non*-medical, perfective interventions. With regard to attempts to correct some *aesthetic* defect — for example, through orthodontic braces or minor cosmetic surgery — it is generally accepted not only that people can consent to such interventions for themselves, but that parents, or others who have special responsibility for children, can consent to such interventions on behalf of children, as they are regarded as in the children's interests.

However, it is generally believed that strangers — for example, the State — are not similiarly entitled to intervene on children in non-therapeutic ways. If this belief is justified, it might be inferred from this that perfective germ-line interventions would be immoral, assuming they were ever feasible, since we do not have the kind of responsibility for our remote descendants which we have for ourselves and our children. While we may engage in medicine and preventive medicine, such as vaccination, for the benefit of strangers including future generations, this is a different matter from attempting to influence strangers in some *perfective* way which supplements or bypasses human teleology.[39]

## *'Perfective'* interventions on children by parents

Even where parents are attempting to influence only their own children, it can be argued that parents should do this, where possible, through the normal environmental channels — for example, through feeding their children, talking to them, playing with them, and so on. If we consider a benefit such as intelligence, it seems intuitively better to *develop* a child's intelligence through early stimulation, rather than to attempt to increase it through genetic or other 'mechanical' interventions (even if these are eventually followed by playing, talking, etc.).

There is nothing wrong with attempting to influence a child by giving him or her an exceptionally favourable environment. Indeed, the environmental side of child development is necessarily 'open-ended': the child is constituted so as to respond to an environment which will be favourable in certain respects, but whose exact characteristics and *degree* of favourability are not specified. However, in attempting to provide the child with a favourable environment, parents should be careful not to control the child in inappropriate ways. They should remember that the child is not theirs to manipulate at will, and that he or she will have *individual* areas of strength and weakness which need to be developed, in addition to those areas which the parents are most interested in seeing developed in him or her.

If we turn from environmental interactions with children to genetic interventions on children, the risk of seeing the child as mere 'raw material' for the parent's plans is surely greater. For mechanical interventions intended to heighten capacities do not involve a mere *response* to *selected existing potential* of the child, but an *amendment* of existing potential of the child. Such interventions are something which *happens* to the child, rather than something the child *does* in a certain environment (whether consciously or unconsciously). Unnecessary interventions which do not themselves involve the child's own activity may encourage the parents to think of the child as something they control, rather than as someone who is in various ways responsible for his or her own fulfilment.

In short, the normal ways of promoting human well-being, including those involving interpersonal co-operation, should be chosen where possible as more respectful of human teleology, and in this way more appropriate to the kind of being we are. In particular, the parental role of nurture, socialization and education is a role distinctive of human beings. To replace or supplement this role, without necessity, by the technical 'fix' of genetic intervention would at least sometimes be unjustified, and conducive to further acts of parental manipulation.

A desire on the part of parents to carry out non-therapeutic interventions on their children may indicate a 'producer's' or 'consumer's' attitude to children, of a kind we have identified in the context of *in vitro* fertilization.[40] If the parents are obsessively concerned with some positive feature it may be that their concern is not to *benefit* the child, but to have the child meet their own personal specifications. In any event, it is doubtful whether a parent could be said to accept his or her child as a gift if *none* of the child's capacities – even in the absence of pathology – was accepted as a 'given' to be developed rather than amended or improved-on.

## *Positive and negative genetic interventions: the responsibility of parents*

While it is widely recognized that at least some non-therapeutic interventions on children involve a 'consumer's' attitude to children, it is less widely recognized that a far more harmful form of this attitude can be seen in the widespread use of prenatal screening. What is absent in either case is what should be an integral feature of the parent-child relationship – an attitude according to which the child is seen as a person equal in dignity to the parents, who is to be welcomed and cared for not as a wanted possession, but for his or her own sake. To abort an existing child due to the presence of some negative trait would appear to involve at least as 'consumerist' an attitude as the obsessive pursuit of positive traits for one's child by genetic or other interventions[41].

As negative genetic interventions are a much more likely outcome of advances in genetic knowledge than positive genetic interventions, it is important to recognize how far some applications of this knowledge are divorced from a view of children as gifts to be accepted unconditionally. Parents are, we have argued, responsible for welcoming every child they may conceive. While this is compatible with attempts to benefit the child either by curing defects or by a limited range of perfective (in practice, non-genetic) interventions, it is not compatible with prenatal selection, or with putting the child to a degree of risk not warranted by the degree and likelihood of benefit.

# 9

# Conclusion: Permissible forms of genetic intervention

Doctors and other health professionals who support the approach to genetic interventions we have outlined will find themselves faced with problems of conscience in dealing with patients and with colleagues who reject this approach. It will be particularly difficult for those who are working in the area of clinical genetics to avoid complicity in the wrongful decisions of others. A doctor may never *intentionally* help his or her patient do something immoral, and should also strive to avoid *unintentionally* helping his or her patient do something immoral – for example, engage in prenatal selection or some unjustified genetic intervention.

However, doctors may, of course, offer their patients forms of treatment which respect their human dignity and the dignity of their children. Such treatments may include somatic therapy, which (as explained above) we regard as morally equivalent to other forms of experimental therapy. *In principle* such acceptable treatments could include germ-line gene therapy; however, in practice, germ-line therapy is likely to involve one or more of various morally unacceptable elements: use of *in vitro* fertilization or similar techniques, experimentation on embryos in the course of developing the therapy, discarding of embryos and abortion of foetuses on whom the therapy is unsuccessful, and the causing of excessive risks to the subject and to his or her descendants.

In contrast, *screening* of gametes – or at least, screening of ova followed by replacement[42] of normal ova and marital intercourse – is far more likely to be morally acceptable than *genetic interventions* on gametes or on embryos. Such a screening procedure would not only escape the moral problems attached to germ-line interventions, but would be likely to be technically simpler. The development of such a procedure would be extremely helpful to those who wish to secure the health of their offspring, while respecting their own dignity and the dignity and life of each child. In addition, as such a procedure might well be safer and simpler than alternative procedures, it could be regarded as helpful even by those who did not share this moral perspective. There is therefore a challenge to doctors and scientists who do share this moral perspective to develop this and all other procedures in which human life and the dignity of human procreation is respected.

In the meantime, those faced with the possibility of having children with genetic disorders should be encouraged to make decisions which are consistent with responsible parenthood, including respect for human life. Those who are already parents of disabled children, whether born or unborn, should be supported by society in accepting and caring for their children. Those who decide, for good reasons, to accept the possibility of conceiving children with genetic disorders should be similarly supported, and should not be subjected to social disapproval.

Finally, those who decide, again for good reasons, to seek to avoid the conception of children with genetic disorders can and should commit themselves to recognizing the value of the lives of existing people with those disorders. For while such disorders are in themselves undesirable, so as to justify our efforts to treat and prevent them, it must be remembered that the lives of the disabled have the basic worth of any human life.

# Appendix A:
# Somatic Gene Therapy and Germ Line Gene Therapy: Legal Issues – Mr John Duddington

*Somatic gene therapy*

The main issue here seems to be consent. If the person (the patient) does not consent to the course of treatment, then an action could be brought in tort for trespass to the person for negligence. The law requires that not only should sufficient information be given to enable the competent patient to understand the nature of the treatment proposed but also to explain the implications of the procedure (*Sidaway v Bethlem Royal Hospital Governors* [1985]). However, Lord Bridge pointed out in *Sidaway* that there is no legal duty to specifically warn a patient of all the risks inherent in treatment offered. The court in *Sidaway* approved of the *Bolam* principle that, in effect, the doctor has a duty to warn of risks in cases where the normal practice of the medical profession would be to warn, but this was by implication disapproved by the High Court of Australia in *Rogers v Whitaker* [1993] where it was held that relevant factors in deciding whether information should be disclosed *included* the patient's temperament, health *and* the patient's own desire for information. Thus if a patient, as in this case, is particularly concerned about a risk of a particular consequence, *but* the doctor fails to warn of this *and* this consequence *does* materialise then there could be liability for negligence.

Accordingly the law does seem to be moving towards a higher duty to disclose risks in treatment and this seems to be particularly relevant in relation to new techniques such as somatic gene therapy.

### Germ Line Gene Therapy

The legal problem here seems to be that as a result of this treatment, injury could be caused to descendants of the patient with the possibility of an action for negligence resulting. In such a case a plaintiff would need to establish the existence of a duty of care which, in the present state of the law, would require consideration of:—

(a) was any harm resulting from the breach of duty reasonably forseeable? and
(b) if so, what considerations are relevant to the imposition of a duty of care in novel situations such as these?
(See Lord Keith in *Murphy v Brentwood DC 1990* and *Brennan J. in Sutherland Shire Council v Heyman* [1985]).

Thus it is possible, although not necessarily probable, that there could be liability in a case resulting from injury from germ-line gene therapy.

One argument in favour of imposing a duty is that the law does, in some circumstances, already recognise a right of action by a child for damage suffered before it was conceived: S1 (3) of the Vaccine Damage Payments Act 1979 allows a child to claim compensation where that child has been born severely disabled as a result of a vaccination against particular diseases given to the child's mother before the child's birth. Furthermore, the Congenital Disabilities (Civil Liability) Act 1976 gives a right of action where the child was born disabled as a result of an occurrence before its birth (not just during pregnancy) although the Act is restricted to cases where the occurrence affected the child's parents and not any remoter case (S1 (4) provides that the Act does *not* apply where the parents actually *knew* of the particular risk). (See above discussion). It should be noted that in *McKay v Essex A.H.A.* [1982] the Court of Appeal, obiter, denied the possibility of an action for wrongful life (i.e.: that the plaintiff should never have been born) resulting from this Act. However, an action brought for damages for loss sustained due to the handicap with which the plaintiff was born could succeed.

Three further points:

(a) **Confidentiality**
It would seem that it would be a breach of the equitable obligation of confidence for information to be disclosed that a person has been subject to germ-line gene therapy or that he or she is a descendant of such a person. Such a duty has been held to arise 'whenever it is unconscionable for a person who has received (confidential) information ... subsequently to reveal that information' (*Stephens v Avery* 1988) and it has been held that it need not be shown that detriment (e.g. damage) resulted from such revelation (X v Y 1988).

(b) **The Human Fertilisation and Embryology Act 1990** does not seem to refer to gene therapy. S.3 provides that a licence is required for bringing about the creation of, or keeping and using, an embryo, but this does not refer to genes. Indeed, the Committee on the Ethics of Gene

Therapy, which reported in 1991, recognised the need for a supervisory body in this area (para 6.1) which would clearly not be necessary if these activities were covered by the Human Fertilisation and Embryology Authority, established under the 1990 Act.

(c) **Consent**

What was said above about consent in relation to somatic gene therapy is clearly relevant here but there is the special issue of the extent to which consent can be given on behalf of those as yet unborn by, for example, their parents. It may be that such consent could be given if, in the existing state of knowledge, it could be said that such treatment appeared to be in the patient's best interests (see e.g. Re F [1989]).

# Appendix B:
# Extracts from Vatican Documents on Disability and Clinical Genetics

## *The Holy See, Statement for the International Year of Disabled Persons (4 March, 1981)*\*

[...] Indeed, on reflection one may say that a disabled person, with the limitations and sufferings that he or she suffers in body and faculties, emphasizes the mystery of the human being with all its dignity and nobility. When we are faced with a disabled person we are shown the hidden frontiers of human existence, and we are impelled to approach this mystery with respect and love.

[...] The quality of a society and a civilization is measured by the respect shown to the weakest of its members. A perfect technological society which only allowed fully functional members and which neglected, institutionalized or, what is worse, eliminated those who did not measure up to this standard or who were unable to carry out a useful role, would have to be considered as radically unworthy of man however economically successful it might be. Such a society would in fact be tainted by a sort of discrimination no less worthy of condemnation than racial discrimination; it would be

\*English text in *Origins*, 7 May, 1981.

discrimination by the strong and 'healthy' against the weak and the sick. It must be clearly affirmed that a disabled person is one of us, a sharer in the same humanity. By recognizing and promoting that person's dignity and rights we are recognizing and promoting our own dignity and our rights [...]

Developments in science and medicine have enabled us today to discover in the fetus some defects which can give rise to future malformations and deficiencies. The impossibility at present of providing a remedy for them by medical means has led some to propose and even to practise the suppression of the fetus. This conduct springs from an attitude of pseudohumanism, which compromises the ethical order of objective values and must be rejected by upright consciences. It is a form of behaviour which if it were applied at a different age would be considered gravely anti-human. Furthermore, the deliberate failure to provide assistance or any act which leads to the suppression of the newborn disabled person represents a breach not only of medical ethics but also of the fundamental and inalienable right to life.

One cannot at whim dispose of human life by claiming an arbitrary power over it. Medicine loses its title of nobility when instead of attacking disease, it attacks life; in fact prevention should be against the illness, not against life. One can never claim that one wishes to bring comfort to a family by suppressing one of its members. The respect, the dedication, the time and means required for the care of handicapped persons, even those whose mental faculties are gravely affected, is the price that a society should generously pay in order to remain truly human.

A consequence of a clear affirmation of this point is the duty to undertake more extensive and thorough research in order to overcome the causes of disabilities. Certainly much has been done in recent years in this field, but much more remains to be done. Scientists have the noble task of placing their skill and their studies at the service of bettering the quality and defense of human life. Present developments in the fields of genetics, fetology, perinatology, biochemistry and neurology, to mention only some disciplines, permit us to foster the hope of noticeable progress.

[...] it is necessary to take into account the decisive importance which lies in the help to be offered at the moment that parents make the painful discovery that one of their children is handicapped. The trauma which derives from this can be so profound and can cause such a strong crisis that it shakes their whole system of values.

The lack of early assistance or adequate support in this phase can have very unfortunate consequences for both the parents and the disabled person. For this reason one should not rest content with only making the diagnosis and then leaving the parents abandoned. Isolation and rejection by society could lead them to refuse to accept or, God forbid, to reject their disabled child. It is necessary therefore for families to be given great understanding and sympathy by the community and to receive from associations and public powers adequate assistance from the beginning of the discovery of the disability of one of their members.

*Pope John Paul II, 'Biological Experimentation' (Address to Participants in the Week of Study Sponsored by the Pontifical Academy of Sciences, October 23, 1982)\**

[...] It is also to be hoped, with reference to your activities, that the new techniques of modification of the genetic code,

\* In *The Pope Speaks*, 28: no.1, 1983.

in particular cases of genetic chromosomic diseases, will be a motive of hope for the great number of people affected by those maladies.

[...] The research of modern biology gives hope that the transfer and mutations of genes can ameliorate the condition of those who are affected by chromosomic diseases; in this way the smallest and weakest of human beings can be cured during their intrauterine life or in the period immediately after birth [...]

## Pope John Paul II, 'The Ethics of Genetic Manipulation' (Address to the World Medical Association, October 29, 1983)*

[...] A strictly therapeutic intervention, having the objective of healing various maladies – such as those stemming from chromosomic deficiencies – will be considered in principle as desirable, provided that it tends to real promotion of the personal well-being of man, without harming his integrity or worsening his life conditions.

[...] But here the question rebounds. It is really of great interest to know whether an intervention upon the genetic store, exceeding the bounds of the therapeutic in the strict sense, is morally acceptable as well. For this to be so, it is necessary for several conditions to be respected and certain premises to be accepted.

[...] in the body and through the body, one touches the person itself, in its concrete reality. Respecting the dignity of man consequently comes down to safeguarding this identity of man *corpore et anima unus* (one in body and soul) as Vatican

*In *Origins*, 17 Nov, 1983.

Council 11 says (*Gaudium et Spes*, 14). It is on the basis of this anthropological view that the fundamental criteria have to be found for making decisions if it is a question of interventions not strictly therapeutic, for example, interventions aimed at improving the human biological condition.

In particular, this kind of intervention must not offer harm to the origin of human life, that is procreation linked not only with the biological but also the spiritual union of the parents, united by the bond of marriage. Such an intervention must consequently respect the fundamental dignity of mankind and the common biological nature which lies at the basis of liberty; respect, consisting in avoidance of manipulations tending to modify the genetic store and to create groups of different people, at the risk of provoking fresh marginalizations in society.

For the rest, the fundamental attitudes inspiring the intervention we refer to should not derive from a racist, materialist mentality, aimed at a human happiness which is really reductive. Man's dignity transcends his biological condition.

Genetic manipulation becomes arbitrary and unjust when it reduces life to an object, when it forgets that it has to do with a human subject, capable of intelligence and liberty, and worthy of respect, whatever its limitations may be; or when genetic manipulation treats the human subject in terms of criteria not founded on the integral reality of the human person, at the risk of doing damage to his dignity. In this case it exposes man to the caprice of others, by depriving him of his autonomy.

All scientific and technical progress whatever must therefore keep the greatest respect for moral values, which constitute a safeguard of the dignity of the human person. And since, in the order of medical values, life is man's supreme and most radical good, there is need for a fundamental principle: First prevent any damage, then seek and pursue the good.

To tell the truth, the expression 'genetic manipulation' remains ambiguous and ought to become the object of genuine moral discernment, for on the one hand it covers adventurous attempts aimed at promoting I know not what superman, and on the other hand salutary efforts aimed at correcting anomalies, such as certain hereditary maladies [...]

### Pope John Paul II, 'Society must protect embryos' (Address to a working party on the legal and ethical aspects of the Human Genome Project, November 20, 1993)*

[...] The human person is not defined according to his present or future activity nor obliged to become what is glimpsed of him in the genome, but according to the essential qualities of his being, the capacities connected with his very nature. From the moment of fertilization, a new being cannot be reduced to its genetic inheritance, which are its biological basis and which hold the promise of life for the subject.

[...] Consequently, to use an embryo as a pure object of analysis or experimentation is to attack the dignity of the person and the human race. Indeed, no one has the right to determine the threshold of humanity for an individual being, which would amount to claiming for himself an inordinate power over his fellow man.

Therefore at no moment in its development can the embryo be the subject of tests that are not beneficial, or of experimentation that would inevitably lead to its destruction or mutilation or irreversibly damage it, for man's nature itself would be mocked and wounded. The genetic inheritance is a treasure

*In *L'Osservatore Romano*, 1 Dec, 1993.

that belongs or could belong to a unique being who has the right to life and integral human growth. Thoughtless manipulations of gametes or embryos, which consist in transforming the specific sequences of the genome that bear the traits proper to the species and the individual, make humanity run the serious risk of genetic mutations that will necessarily alter the spiritual and physical integrity not only of the human beings on which these alterations are made but even more on individuals in future generations.

If it is not ordered to his good, experimentation on man, which first seems an achievement in the area of knowledge, risks leading to the degradation of the authentic dignity and value of what is human. In fact, the moral criteria for research is always man in his physical and spiritual being. The ethical sense implies not being willing to engage in research that would offend his human dignity or hamper his overall growth. This is not however to condemn researchers to ignorance; they are invited to redouble their ingenuity. With a keen sense of what a man is, they will be able to find new paths of knowledge and carry out the invaluable service expected from them by the human community.

# Glossary

**adenosine deaminase (ADA) deficiency**
A genetic disorder caused by the lack of the gene product adenosine deaminase and involving an abnormality of bone marrow cells leading to recurrent infections.

**alleles**
Alternative forms of a gene which may occupy a particular locus on a chromosome.

**amino acids**
The building blocks of proteins.

**antigen**
A substance having the power to elicit antibody formation by cells and to react specifically with the antibody so produced.

**autosomes**
Chromosomes other than sex chromosomes.

**base**
Here, one of four compounds, cytosine, adenine, thymine and guanine (C, A, T and G) which are the components of DNA which enable it to carry genetic information.

**chromosomes**
Bundles of DNA found in pairs in body cells, but singly in gametes.

**chronic granulomatous disease**
A disease characterized by repeated infections with granuloma and abscess formation.

**cystic fibrosis**
An autosomal recessive disease, characterized by abnormally thick mucus which tends to obstruct the organ ducts, resulting in a variety of clinical problems.

**DNA (deoxyribonucleic acid)**
The chemical of which genes are made.

**dominant**
Describes the state of affairs when a gene inherited from one parent overrides the expression of the gene on the other chromosome.

**Down's syndrome**
A genetic disorder accompanied by learning difficulty, resulting most commonly from the possession of three instead of two copies of chromosome 21. Due to the gross nature of the chromosomal defect, Down's syndrome is perhaps less likely than other genetic conditions to be amenable to gene therapy.

**gamete**
A reproductive cell: sperm in males, ova in females.

**gene**
A sequence of DNA which codes for one polypeptide. The basic unit of heredity by which traits are passed on from one generation to the next.

**gene expression**
The production by a cell of the polypeptide for which the gene codes.

**genotype**
An individual's genetic constitution.

**germ-line cells**
Ova or sperm or their precursors, including cells set aside in the embryonic sex organs.

**haemophilia**
A sex-linked recessive disorder characterised by excessive bleeding due to defective production of a protein required for blood clotting. Symptoms can be successfully contained with modern haematological treatments.

**Human Genome Project**
Co-operative work by scientists in different countries on the location of genes on chromosomes and the definition of their chemical structures.

**Huntington's Chorea**
A dominant genetic disorder in which, during adult life, there is worsening involuntary movement and progressive dementia, and which leads eventually to the death of the patient.

**karyotype**
An individual's set of chromosomes.

**lipid vesicles (lipoproteins)**
Fatty bubbles which can be used as vectors

**locus**
The place on a chromosome occupied by a gene.

**lymphocytes**
A type of white blood cell, important in immunity.

**meiosis**
The cell division by which gametes, containing only one from each pair of chromosomes (i.e., 23 chromosomes) are formed from cells containing the full complement of 46 chromosomes.

**mitochondria**
DNA-bearing structures outside the cell nucleus

**mitosis**
Somatic cell division resulting in the formation of two cells, each with the same chromosomal complement as the parent cell.

**(Duchenne) muscular dystrophy**
A sex-linked recessive disorder characterized by progressive weakness and degeneration of muscle fibres, usually leading to death in late adolescence.

**phenotype**
The expression of the genotype in an individual's structure or physiology.

**polypeptide**
The chain of amino acids which comprises part or all of a protein.

**receptor**
A structure or site on the surface or interior of a cell which binds with substances such as hormones or antigens.

**recessive**
Describes the state of affairs when a gene exercises little or no outward effect unless it is present in both chromosomes; i.e., inherited from both parents.

**replication**
The process whereby DNA makes copies of itself when a cell divides.

**RNA (ribonucleic acid)**
A nucleic acid formed on a DNA template and taking part in the synthesis of polypeptides. Messenger RNA or mRNA is the means whereby the recipe for a polypeptide encoded in DNA which is contained in the nucleus of a cell is transcribed and carried outside the nucleus to the place in the cell where proteins are synthesized.

**sex-linked disorder**
A genetic disorder carried on one of the sex chromosomes, and so affecting only one sex.

**somatic cell**
Any cell of the body except a germ-line cell. Changes to somatic cells affect only the individual whose cells they are.

**spermatogonia**
The precursors of sperm.

**teleology**
Goal-directedness; here, a goal-directed human function.

**transcription**
The process whereby the genetic information contained in DNA is transferred to the messenger RNA as it is being synthesized.

**translation**
The process whereby the genetic information present in mRNA directs the order of the amino acids during the synthesis of protein.

**vector**
A delivery system for inserting a gene into a cell.

# Bibliography

'The ADA human gene treated', *Human Gene Therapy*, vol. 1, 1990, pp. 327–9.
Alberts, B., Bray, D., Lewis, J., Raff, M., Roberts, K. and Watson, J., *Molecular Biology of the Cell (Second Edition)*, New York, 1989.
Alper, J.S., 'Genetic complexity in single gene diseases', *British Medical Journal*, vol. 312, no. 7025, 1996, pp. 196–197.
Archer, L., 'Genetic Engineering and Human Freedom', *Catholic Medical Quarterly*, vol. 41, no. 1, 1990, pp. 6–19.
Ashley, B.M., *Theologies of the Body: Humanist and Christian*, Braintree, Mass., 1985.
Ashley, B.M., and O'Rourke, K.D., *Health Care Ethics: A Theological Analysis (Third Edition)*, St Louis, 1989.
Bankowski, Z., and Capron, A.M.(Eds), *Genetics, Ethics and Human Values: Human Genome Mapping, Genetic Screening and Gene Therapy, Proceedings of the XXIVth CIOMS Round Table Conference*, Council for International Organisations of Medical Sciences, Geneva, 1991.
Beauchamp, T.L., and Childress, J.F., *Principles of Biomedical Ethics (Third Edition)*, Oxford, 1989.

Bednarik, D.P., Mosca, J.D., Raj, N.B., Pitha, P.M., 'Inhibition of human immunodeficiency virus (HIV) replication by HIV-trans-activated alpha 2-interferon', *Proceedings of the National Academy of Sciences*, vol. 86, 1989, pp. 4958–62.

Bishop, J.E., and Waldholz, M., *Genome*, New York, 1990.

Bone, E., 'Genetic Engineering: how far may we go?', *Month* (SNS), vol. 19, no. 11, 1986, pp. 288–295.

Braine, D., 'Human animality: its relevance to the shape of ethics', in D. Braine and H. Lesser (Eds), *Ethics, Technology and Medicine*, Aldershot, 1988, pp. 6–30.

Braine, D., *The Human Person: Animal and Spirit*, London, 1993.

British Medical Association, *Our Genetic Future: The Science amd Ethics of Genetic Technology*, Oxford, 1992.

Buchanon, K., 'The Ultimate Arrogance: genetic engineering and the human future', *New Blackfriars*, vol. 69, no. 812, 1988, pp. 35–44.

Carrington Coutts, M., 'Human Gene Therapy', *Kennedy Institute of Ethics Journal*, vol. 4, no. 1, 1994, pp. 63–82.

Burnet, M., 'Biomedical Research: Changes and Opportunities', in N. Black, D. Boswell, A. Gray, S. Murphy and J. Popay (Eds), *Health and Disease: A Reader*, Milton Keynes, 1984.

Cassidy, J.D., and Pellegrino, E.D., 'A Catholic Perspective on Human Gene Therapy', *International Journal of Bioethics*, vol. 4, no. 1, 1993, pp. 11–18.

Catholic Bishops' Joint Committee on Bioethical Issues, *Submission to the Warnock Committee ('In Vitro Fertilisation: Morality and Public Policy')*, Abingdon, 1983.

Charlesworth, M., 'Human genome analysis and the concept of human nature', in D. Chadwick, G. Bock and

J. Whelan (Eds), *Human Genetic Information: Science, Law and Ethics*, Ciba Foundation Symposium, 1990, pp. 180–198.

Clarke, A. (Ed), *Genetic Counselling: Practice and Principles*, London, 1994.

*Clothier Committee Report on the Ethics of Gene Therapy*, London, 1992.

Coghlan, A., 'Outrage greets patent on designer sperm', *New Scientist*, 9 April, 1994, pp. 4–5.

Cole, A. P., Duddington, J., Jessiman, I., and Williamson, J., 'The Human Genome Project and Gene Therapy: Clinical and ethical considerations', *Catholic Medical Quarterly*, vol. 42, no. 4, 1992, pp. 24–28.

Congregation for the Doctrine of the Faith, *Instruction on Respect for Human Life in its Origin and on the Dignity of Procreation (Donum Vitae)*, Vatican City, 1987.

Cummings, M. R., 'Gene Therapy: Actualities and Possibilities', in R. Smith (Ed), *The Twenty Fifth Anniversary of Vatican II: A Look Back and A Look Ahead*, Braintree, Mass., 1990, pp. 64–77.

*The Danish Council of Ethics Second Annual Report, 1989, Protection of human gametes, fertilized ova, embryos and fetuses*, Copenhagen, 1990.

Danks, D. M., 'Human Gene Therapy: The Present and the Foreseeable Future', *St Vincent's Bioethics Centre Newsletter, Supplement: Genetic Engineering*, vol. 10, no. 1, 1992.

Elliot, R., 'Identity and the Ethics of Gene Therapy', *Bioethics*, vol. 7, no. 1, 1993, pp. 27–40.

Emery, A.E.H., Mueller, R. F., *Elements of Medical Genetics (Seventh Edition)*, London, 1988.

Finchasm, J.R.S., and Ravetz, J. R., in collaboration with a working party of the Council for Science and Society, *Genetically Engineered Organisms: Benefits and Risks*, Oxford, 1991.

Finnis, J., *Natural Law and Natural Rights*, Oxford, 1980.

Fletcher, J.C., 'Moral Problems and Ethical Issues in Prospective Human Gene Therapy', *Virginia Law Review*, vol. 69, no. 3, pp. 515–46.

Fletcher, J.C., 'Controversies in Research Ethics Affecting the Future of Human Gene Therapy', *Human Gene Therapy*, vol. 1, 1990, pp. 307–324.

French Anderson, W., Editorial: 'Uses and Abuses of Human Gene Transfer', *Human Gene Therapy*, vol. 3, 1992, pp. 1–2.

Friedmann, T., 'Some Ethical Implications of Human Gene Therapy', in Z. Bankowski and A. M. Capron (Eds), *Genetics, Ethics and Human Values: Human Genome Mapping, Genetic Screening and Gene Therapy, Proceedings of the XXIVth CIOMS Round Table Conference*, Council for International Organisations of Medical Sciences, Geneva, 1991, pp. 132–138.

*Gene Therapy Advisory Committee First Annual Report*, November 1993–December 1994, 1995.

Gene Therapy in Man, a joint statement by European Medical Research Councils (Austria, Denmark, Finland, France, The Netherlands, Norway, Spain, Sweden, Switzerland, the United Kingdom and West Germany), *Lancet*, no. 8597, 1988, pp. 1271–1272.

German Enquete Commission, 'A Report from Germany', *Bioethics*, vol. 2, no.3, 1988, pp. 254–263.

Glover, J. et al., *Fertility and the Family: The Glover Report on*

Reproductive Technologies to the European Commission, London, 1989.

Gormally, L., 'The Status of the Human Genome', *Dolentium Hominum*, no. 28, 1995, pp. 27–32.

Gormally, L. (Ed), *Euthanasia, Clinical Practice and the Law*, London, 1994.

Gormally, L., 'The Practice of Medicine and the Need for Moral Consensus', in J. Glasa (Ed), *Contemporary Problems of Medical Ethics in Central Europe*, Bratislava, 1992, pp.15–24.

Grisez, G., *The Way of the Lord Jesus. Volume 2: Living a Christian Life*, Quincy, Illinois, 1993.

Grisez, G., Boyle, J., and Finnis, J., 'Practical Principles, Moral Truth and Ultimate Ends', *American Journal of Jurisprudence*, vol. 32, 1987, pp. 99–151.

Guild of Catholic Doctors Submission to the British Medical Association Genetic Engineering Working Party, *Catholic Medical Quarterly*, vol. 41, no. 1, 1990, pp. 37–39.

Harris, J., 'Is Gene Therapy A Form of Eugenics?', *Bioethics*, vol. 7, no. 2/3, 1993, pp. 178–187.

Holtug, N., 'Human Gene Therapy: Down the Slippery Slope?', *Bioethics*, vol. 7, no. 5, 1993, pp. 402–419.

Hoose, B., 'Gene Therapy: Where to Draw the Line', *Human Gene Therapy*, vol. 1, 1990, pp. 299–306.

Huber, B.E., Richards, C.A., and Krenitsky, T.A., 'Retroviral-mediated gene therapy for the treatment of hepatocellular carcinoma: an innovative approach for cancer therapy', *Proceedings of the National Academy of Sciences*, vol. 88, 1991, pp. 8039–43.

John Paul II, Message for the International Year of Disabled

Persons, March 4, 1981, in *Origins*, 7 May 1981, pp. 747–750.

John Paul II, Apostolic Exhortation *Familiaris Consortio*, *Acta Apostolicae Sedis* 73, 1981.

John Paul II, Address to a Meeting of the Pontifical Academy of Sciences, October 23, 1982, *Acta Apostolicae Sedis* 75, 1983.

John Paul II, Discourse to those taking part in the 35th General Assembly of the World Medical Association, October 29, 1983, *Acta Apostolicae Sedis* 76, 1984.

John Paul II, Address to a Working Party on the Legal and Ethical Aspects of the Human Genome Project, November 20, 1993, *L'Osservatore Romano*, 1 December, 1993.

John Paul II, Encyclical Letter *Evangelium Vitae*, March 25, 1995, Vatican City.

Joint Ethico-Medical Committee of the Catholic Union of Great Britain and the Guild of Catholic Doctors, Submission to the Committee on the Ethics of Gene Therapy, *Catholic Medical Quarterly*, vol. 41, no. 2, 1990, pp. 79–84.

Jones, S., *The Language of the Genes: Biology, History and the Evolutionary Future*, London, 1994.

Juengst, E.T., 'Germ-Line Gene Therapy: Back to Basics', *Human Gene Therapy*, vol. 3, 1992, pp. 45–49.

Kahn, J., 'Genetic Harm: Bitten By The Body That Keeps You?', *Bioethics*, vol. 3, no. 4, 1991, pp. 289–308.

Keenan, J.F., 'What Is Morally New in Genetic Manipulation?', *Human Gene Therapy*, vol. 1, 1990, pp. 289–298.

Kevles, D.J., *In the Name of Eugenics: Genetics and the Uses of Human Heredity*, Berkeley and Los Angeles, 1985.

Kevles, D.J., and Hood, L., *The Code of Codes*, Cambridge, 1992.

Knowles, M. et al, 'A controlled study of adenoviral-vector-mediated gene transfer in the nasal epithelium of patients with cystic fibrosis', *New England Journal of Medicine*, vol. 333, no. 13, 1995, pp. 823–831.

Latchman, D. (Ed), *From Genetics to Gene Therapy*, Oxford, 1994.

Leiden, J., 'Gene Therapy – Promise, Pitfalls and Prognosis', *New England Journal of Medicine*, vol. 333, no. 13, 1995, pp. 871–873.

Lever, A.M.L., 'Gene therapy for genetic, malignant, metabolic and infectious disease', *Proceedings of the Royal College of Physicians Edinburgh*, vol. 23, 1993, pp. 424–427.

Lewontin, R.C., *The Doctrine of DNA: Biology as Ideology*, Harmondsworth, 1993.

Macer, D.R.J., *Shaping Genes: Ethics, Law and Science Using Genetic Technology in Medicine and Agriculture*, Christchurch, 1990.

Marshall, E., 'Gene Therapy's Growing Pains', *Science*, vol. 269, 1995, pp. 1050–1055.

McMullan, G., and Andrews, K., *Manipulating Life: An ethical and legal response to Human Gene Therapy*, St Vincent's Bioethics Centre, Melbourne, 1988.

*The Medical Research Council of Canada Guidelines for Research on Somatic Cell Gene Therapy in Humans*, 1990.

Mendell, J. R. et al, 'Myoblast transfer in the treatment of Duchenne's Muscular Dystrophy', *New England Journal of Medicine*, vol. 333, no. 13, 1995, pp. 832–838.

Moraczewski, A., 'The Human Genome Project and the Catholic Church', *International Journal of Bioethics*, vol. 12, no. 4, 1991, pp. 229–234.

Moraczewski, A. (Ed), *Genetic Medicine and Engineering: Ethical and Social Dimensions*, Catholic Health Association of the

United States and Pope John XXIII Medical-Moral Research and Education Centre, St. Louis, 1983.

Munson, R., and Davis, L.H., 'Germ-Line Gene Therapy and the Medical Imperative', *Kennedy Institute of Ethics Journal*, vol. 2, no. 2, 1992, pp. 137–158.

Miyanohara, A., Sharkey, M.F., Witztum, J.L., Steinberg, D., and Friedmann, T., 'Efficient expression of retroviral vector-transduced human low density lipoprotein (LDL) receptor in LDL receptor-deficient rabbit fibroblasts in vitro', *Proceedings of the National Academy of Sciences*, vol.85, 1988, pp. 6538–42.

Nossal, G.J.V., and Coppel, R.L., *Reshaping Life: Key Issues in Genetic Engineering (Second Edition)*, Cambridge, 1989.

Paul VI, Encyclical Letter *Humanae Vitae*, *Acta Apostolicae Sedis* 60, 1968.

Pembrey, M., *Genetics: A Simple Guide*, London, 1994.

Persson, I., 'Genetic Therapy, Identity and The Person-Regarding Reasons', *Bioethics*, vol. 9, no.1, 1995, pp. 16–31.

Pius XII, Allocution to midwives, October 29, 1951, in *The Human Body: Papal Teachings*, Boston, 1960, pp. 163–165.

Pius XII, Allocution to those attending the 'Primum Symposium Geneticae Medicae', September 7, 1953, in *The Human Body: Papal Teachings*, Boston, 1960, pp. 256–258, 260.

Pius XII, Allocution to the Members of the 7th International Congress on Blood Transfusion, September 5, 1958, *L'Osservatore Romano*, September 10, 1958.

Pius XII, Allocution to the 7th International Congress of Haematology, September 12, 1958, *Acta Apostolicae Sedis* 50, 1958.

Pyeritz, R.E., 'Medical Genetics', in S. Schroeder, M. Krupp, L. Therney and S. McPhee (Eds), *Current Medical Diagnosis and Treatment*, Norwalk, Connecticut, 1991, pp. 1174–1190.

*Report of the Office of Science and Technology Assessment of the US Congress*, 1984.

Resnik, D., 'Debunking the Slippery Slope Argument Against Human Germ-Line Gene Therapy', *Journal of Medicine and Philosophy*, vol. 19, no. 1, 1994, pp. 23–40.

Rifkin, J., *Who Should play God? The Artificial Creation of Life and What it Means for the Future of the Human Race*, New York, 1977.

Rose, S., Lewontin, R.C., and Kamin, L.J., *Not in Our Genes: Biology, Ideology and Human Nature*, Harmondsworth, 1988.

Rosenfeld, M.A., Yoshimura, K., Trapnell, B.C. *et al.*, 'In vivo transfer of the human cystic fibrosis transmembrane conductance regulator gene to the airway epithelium', *Cell*, vol. 68, 1992, pp. 143–55.

Rubenstein, D.S., Thomasma, D.C., Schon, E.A., and Zinaman, M.J., 'Germ-Line Therapy to Cure Mitochondrial Disease: Protocol and Ethics of In Vitro Ovum Nuclear Transplantation', *Cambridge Quarterly of Healthcare Ethics*, vol. 4, no. 3, 1995, pp. 316–339.

Sacred Congregation for the Doctrine of the Faith, *Declaration on Procured Abortion (Quaestio de Abortu Procurato)*, Acta Apostolicae Sedis 66, 1974.

Sass, H.M., 'A Critique of the Enquete Commission's Report on Gene Therapy', *Bioethics*, vol. 2, no. 3, 1988, pp. 264–275.

*Science and Technology Committee Third Report ('Human Genetics: The Science and Its Consequences')*, 1995.

Sutton, A., *Prenatal Diagnosis: Confronting the Ethical Issues*, London, 1990.

Sutton, A., 'The new gene technology and the difference between getting rid of illness and altering people', *European Journal of Genetics in Society*, vol. 1, no. 1, 1995, pp. 12–20.

Suzuki, D., and Knudtson, P., *Genethics: The Ethics of Engineering Life*, London, 1989.

Wachter, M.A.M., 'Ethical Aspects of Human Germ-Line Gene Therapy', *Bioethics*, vol. 7, no. 2/3, 1993, pp. 166–177.

von Wartburg, W.P., 'Health Policy Aspects of Gene Therapy', in Z. Bankowski and A. M. Capron (Eds), *Genetics, Ethics and Human Values: Human Genome Mapping, Genetic Screening and Gene Therapy. Proceedings of the XXIVth CIOMS Round Table Conference*, Council for International Organisations of Medical Sciences, Geneva, 1991, pp. 162–177.

Watt, H., 'Genetic Intervention and the Good of Human Beings', *Catholic Medical Quarterly*, vol. 44, no. 1, 1993, pp. 17–21.

Wills, C., *Exons, Introns and Talking Genes: The Science Behind the Human Genome Project*, Oxford, 1992.

Wills, C., *The Wisdom of the Genes: New Pathways in Evolution*, Oxford, 1991.

Wingerson, L., *Mapping our Genes: The Genome Project and the Future of Medicine*, New York, 1991.

World Council of Churches Subunit on Church and Society, *Biotechnology: Its Challenges to the Churches and the World*, Geneva, 1989.

Wyngaarden, J. B., 'Current Status of Science of Human

Genetics', *International Journal of Bioethics*, vol. 4, no. 2, 1993, pp. 103–110.

Zimmerman, B.K., 'Human Germ-Line Therapy: The Case for Its Development and Use', *The Journal of Medicine and Philosophy*, vol. 6, no. 6, pp. 593–612.

Zohar, N.J., 'Commentary on Khan's "Genetic Harm: Bitten By The Body That Keeps You?"', *Bioethics*, vol. 5, no. 4, 1991, pp. 275–288.

# Notes

1. The definition of 'disease' which we will use in this Report is that given in Dorlands Medical Dictionary (26th edition): 'A deviation from or interruption of a normal structure or function of any part, organ or system (or combination thereof) of the body that is manifested by a characteristic set of symptoms and signs and whose aetiology, pathology and prognosis may be known or unknown'. 'Normal' here should be understood as 'healthy', and not simply as 'statistically prevalent'.
2. There are many different mutations of the cystic fibrosis gene. Some combinations of mutations are benign, while others will result in cystic fibrosis of varying degrees of severity. Even in the case of a single gene disorder such as cystic fibrosis, it seems that environmental factors or interactions of the cystic fibrosis gene with other genes may be important in influencing the severity of the disease. See Alper, J.S., 'Genetic complexity in single gene diseases', *British Medical Journal*, vol. 312, no. 7025, 1996, pp. 196-197.
3. We acknowledge the help of the following sources in writing this section: Alberts, B., Bray, D., Lewis, J., Raff, M., Roberts, K., and Watson, J., *Molecular Biology of the Cell (Second*

Edition), New York, 1989; Latchman, D.S. (Ed), *From Genetics to Gene Therapy*, Oxford, 1994; *Clothier Committee Report on the Ethics of Gene Therapy*, London, 1992; Pembrey, M., *Genetics: A Simple Guide*, London, 1994.
4. Marshall, E., 'Gene Therapy's Growing Pains', *Science*, vol. 269, 1995, pp. 1050–1055.
5. 'The ADA human gene treated', *Human Gene Therapy*, vol. 1, 1990, pp. 327–9.
6. Marshall, E., 'Gene Therapy's Growing Pains', *Science*, vol. 269, 1995, p. 1051.
7. Rosenfeld, M.A., Yoshimura, K., Trapnell, B.C. et al., 'In vivo transfer of the human cystic fibrosis transmembrane conductance regulator gene to the airway epithelium', *Cell*, vol. 68, 1992, pp. 143–55; Knowles, M. *et al*, 'A controlled study of adenoviral-vector-mediated gene transfer in the nasal epithelium of patients with cystic fibrosis', *New England Journal of Medicine*, vol. 333, no.13, 1995, pp. 823–831.
8. Lever, A.M.L., 'Gene therapy for genetic, malignant, metabolic and infectious disease', *Proceedings of the Royal College of Physicians Edinburgh*, vol. 23, 1993, pp. 424–427.
9. Huber, B.E., Richards, C.A., and Krenitsky, T.A., 'Retroviral-mediated gene therapy for the treatment of hepatocellular carcinoma: an innovative approach for cancer therapy', *Proceedings of the National Academy of Sciences*, vol. 88, 1991, pp. 8039–43.
10. Bednarik, D.P., Mosca, J.D., Raj, N.B., Pitha, P.M., 'Inhibition of human immunodeficiency virus (HIV) replication by HIV-trans-activated alpha 2-interferon', *Proceedings of the National Academy of Sciences*, vol. 86, 1989, pp. 4958–62.
11. Miyanohara, A., Sharkey, M.F., Witztum, J.L., Steinberg, D., and Friedmann, T., 'Efficient expression of retroviral vector-transduced human low density lipoprotein (LDL)

receptor in LDL receptor-deficient rabbit fibroblasts in vitro', *Proceedings of the National Academy of Sciences*, vol.85, 1988, pp. 6538–42.

12. It is defined Catholic teaching that the soul is the 'form' of the body, and that the soul survives death (cf. Council of Vienne, 1312, Denzinger-Shoenmetzer Enchiridion Symbolorum (1965) 902; Lateran Council V, 1513, Denzinger-Shoenmetzer Enchiridion Symbolorum (1965) 1440). However, neither the concept of survival after death, nor the understanding of the soul as the body's 'life-principle' are specifically religious concepts. For a philosophical exploration of the nature of the soul, see David Braine, *The Human Person: Animal and Spirit*, London, 1993.

13. See (for example) Finnis, J., *Natural Law and Natural Rights*, Oxford, 1980, and Grisez, G., Boyle, J., and Finnis, J., 'Practical Principles, Moral Truth and Ultimate Ends', *American Journal of Jurisprudence*, vol. 32, 1987, pp. 99–151.

14. If a human person is a human being with human moral status, and human beings have morally significant interests simply as the kind of being they are, then 'human being' and 'human person' are co-extensive – i.e., human moral status is intrinsic to human beings.

15. Gormally, L. (Ed), *Euthanasia, Clinical Practice and the Law*, London, 1994, pp. 118–119, 124.

16. Paul VI, Encyclical Letter *Humanae Vitae*, *Acta Apostolicae Sedis* 60, 1968.

17. Congregation for the Doctrine of the Faith, *Instruction on Respect for Human Life in its Origin and on the Dignity of Procreation (Donum Vitae)*, Vatican City, 1987.

18. It should be noted that the prohibition of contraception and IVF, which concerns the morally appropriate forms of parenthood and sexual behaviour, is absolute, unlike what are

often mere *prima facie* objections to the disruption or bypassing of bodily systems in other contexts.

19. See the Catholic Bishops' Joint Committee on Bioethical Issues Submission to the Warnock Committee ('In Vitro Fertilisation: Morality and Public Policy'), Abingdon, 1983.

20. To say that a functional defect is now involuntary is not to deny that it may have been caused by voluntary behaviour forseen to cause that defect.

21. For example, the World Health Organisation defined health in 1958 as 'a state of complete physical, mental, and social well-being and not merely the absence of disease or infirmity'.

22. Declaration of Helsinki: Recommendations guiding medical doctors in biomedical research involving human subjects, adopted by the 18th World Medical Assembly, Helsinki, 1964, as revised by the 29th World Medical Assembly, Tokyo, 1979, section 1.5.

23. Pius XII, Allocution to those attending the 'Primum Symposium Geneticae Medicae', September 7, 1953, in *The Human Body: Papal Teachings*, Boston, 1960, pp. 256–258, 260; Pius XII, Allocution to the Members of the 7th International Congress on Blood Transfusion, September 5, 1958, *L'Osservatore Romano*, 10 September, 1958; Pius XII, Allocution to the 7th International Congress of Haematology, September 12, 1958, *Acta Apostolicae Sedis* 50, 1958.

24. Ashley, B.M., O'Rourke, K.D., *Health Care Ethics: A Theological Analysis (Third Edition)*, St Louis, 1989, p. 326.

25. Gormally, L. (Ed), *Euthanasia, Clinical Practice and the Law*, London, 1994, pp. 128–129.

26. Sutton, A., *Prenatal Diagnosis: Confronting the Ethical Issues*, London, 1990, pp. 48–54.

27. Even where the parents do not intend to seek abortion should the child be found to be disabled, invasive techniques of prenatal diagnosis carry the risk of causing either miscarriage or malformations, with no compensatory benefits which could justify causing such risks.

28. It has been suggested that there may be some risk, however slight, of affecting the germ-line as a side-effect of somatic gene therapy. Thus female patients taking part in trials of somatic therapy have been required to use contraception (*Gene Therapy Advisory Committee First Annual Report, November 1993 – December 1994*, 1995, pp. 5–6). Such risks are not specific to somatic gene therapy, as other forms of treatment of individual patients can carry some risk of causing genetic damage to their children, and perhaps even to later generations. We do not, of course, accept the use of contraception, as opposed to natural family planning, as a way of minimizing such risks.

29. For example, the risks to the mother if gene therapy were to be carried out on an unborn child. Here we are envisaging not germ-line therapy on the embryo (discussed in the next section) but somatic therapy performed sufficiently late in pregnancy to affect only the foetus, and not his or her descendants. There are precedents for treatment *in utero*; for example, infusions of red blood cells to treat a child affected by Rhesus incompatibility.

30. This was the recommendation made by the Clothier Committee (*Report of the Committee on the Ethics of Gene Therapy*, London, 1992, para. 7.4).

31. Congregation for the Doctrine of the Faith, *Instruction on Respect for Human Life in its Origin and on the Dignity of Procreation (Donum Vitae)*, Vatican City, 1987; Catholic Bishops' Joint Committee on Bioethical Issues, *Submission to the Warnock*

Committee ('*In Vitro Fertilisation: Morality and Public Policy*'), Abingdon, 1983.

32. By therapy on spermatogonia we do not mean the technique (which has been carried out on experimental animals) by which spermatogonia can be transplanted from one male individual to another. Clearly, if this technique were carried out on humans, the children would not result from the *integral self-giving* of husband and wife, since they would be genetically the children of the donor, not the children of the husband. Similar, though not identical objections can be raised to recent proposals for treating *mitochondrial* genetic diseases: that is, diseases in DNA-bearing structures outside the nucleus itself. It has been suggested that the nucleus from the ovum of the carrier could be transplanted into a donor ovum with healthy mitochondria after the removal of the nucleus of the donor ovum (Rubenstein, D.S., Thomasma, D.C., Schon, E. A., and Zinaman, M. J., 'Germ-Line Therapy to Cure Mitochondrial Disease: Protocol and Ethics of In Vitro Ovum Nuclear Transplantation', *Cambridge Quarterly of Healthcare Ethics*, vol. 4, no. 3, 1995, pp. 316–339). Even assuming that unfertilized ova were used in both cases, and that the 'combination' ovum was then fertilized through normal marital intercourse, the woman who provided the nucleus could not be said to have contributed a *gamete* by an act of *integral bodily self-giving*. The child would, in fact, be confronted with two candidates for the role of biological mother: the provider of the nucleus of one disassembled ovum and the provider of the mitochondria (and other portions) of another.

33. Moreover, genes which are harmful in one respect – and thus potential targets for gene therapy – may be beneficial in another.

34. Here we do not mean to suggest that there are no moral

criteria governing experimentation on animals, but rather, that such moral criteria are different from those governing experimentation on humans.

35. See John Paul II, Encyclical Letter *Evangelium Vitae*, March 25, 1995, Vatican City, esp. para 74, 76, Chapter 1V.

36. Here we are not referring to non-therapeutic interventions such as haircuts, ear-piercing, etc., which either do not involve a loss of function at all, or do not involve a significant or permanent loss of function.

37. John Paul II, addressing the topic of genetic engineering, has condemned interventions which seek to alter traits proper to the human species and to the human individual (see Appendix B).

38. While there will be borderline cases in which it is hard to draw the distinction between perfective and therapeutic interventions, in many cases an intervention will be either clearly therapeutic, or clearly perfective.

39. It may be objected that we seek to benefit future generations in many ways which are not therapeutic − for example, by creating or preserving beautiful buildings, protecting the environment, and so on. However these are changes which involve no more than *environmental input* to *normal human teleology*: to the normal tendency of human beings to appreciate their environment. Future generations are not being brainwashed in some way; there is no bypassing of normal processes involving consciousness and choice. Rather, future generations are being given environmental stimulus of a kind we constantly provide for members of our own generation.

40. Some of the same objections apply to a situation in which parents are not attempting to influence an individual child who exists or will exist, but are attempting, through selection of gametes, to have a child of one kind rather than a different

child of another (healthy) kind. This, in addition to the manipulation of embryos, may be one of the situations envisaged by *Donum Vitae* where it condemns 'attempts to influence chromosomic or genetic inheritance ... aimed at producing human beings selected according to sex or other predetermined qualities.' (Congregation for the Doctrine of the Faith, *Instruction on Respect for Human Life in its Origin and on the Dignity of Procreation (Donum Vitae)*, Vatican City, 1987, para. 1.6). It can be argued that a relationship of *domination* over children is created by an attempt to have one's preferences met with regard to the *features* of one's children – features which (unlike the *timing* of conception) may be a focus of parental attention – and thus of parental satisfaction or dissatisfaction – throughout the child's life. Whether or not it is ever justifiable to attempt to conceive a child of one kind rather than a different child of another (healthy) kind, such attempts would often be found in the context of an attitude of domination over children: an attitude which sees children as something to be created, like consumer goods, for the satisfaction of parents.

41. We recognize that parents who abort for handicap may be sincerely intending to benefit the child, if the handicap is sufficiently serious. However, their action is unjustified, however well-intentioned, as the life of the child has the 'core value' of any human life. For an extended discussion of euthanasiast killing, see Gormally, L. (Ed), *Euthanasia, Clinical Practice and the Law*, London, 1994.

42. We do not exclude the theoretical possibility that ova could also be screened *in situ*.